Raising the Bar at 50 and Older

Fitness Lessons to Energize Your Life

by Lemuel B. Thomas Jr.

Raising the Bar at 50 and Older
Fitness Lessons to Energize Your Life

By: Lemuel B. Thomas Jr.

Author: L.T. Thomas
Editor: Deb Stratas
Photography: Keron Brown
Website: https://www.lemuelthomasfit.com/

ISBN: 978-0-359-25178-0

Acknowledgments

I wish to thank the following people for helping and inspiring me. I am blessed to have all of you in my life.

Felicia – My wife has listened to all my ideas and has helped me to grow into a better person. Thanks for having my back and supporting me in everything I do.

Lemuel 3rd – to my son, for bringing so much joy in my life.

My mother Chassie and my dad Lemuel Sr. for believing in me and having my back. Thank you for fueling my passion for fitness and sports. Thanks for encouraging me in every aspect of life.

My grand mother – Mama Eames thank you for always supporting me and give me your wisdom.

Brothers and sisters – Felicia, Charles, Tar, and Ciara for helping me grow and listening to all my ideas.

Uncle Charles & Aunt Al

Uncle Nield

Aunt Cythinia

Cheyney

Aunt Diane

Uncle Phil

Thanks to all my teachers and coaches for encouraging me.

High School Football Coach – Mr. Bridges & Coach Sanders

Track Coach – Mr. Brown

TABLE OF CONTENT

Chapter One
Introduction

"Even though the future seems far away, it is actually beginning right now."
Mattie Stepanek

Energize, Empower, & Elevate

I want to personally congratulate you for taking the first step to improving your health. The first one is usually the hardest, so it takes courage right from the start. The stories and the advice that I share in this book will guide you to live a healthier and happier? life. I will give you actions that you can apply to empower you on your health and fitness journey. I titled this book Raising the Bar because it's possible for everyone to live a healthy lifestyle. You don't have to be elite to raise the bar. All you have to do is be willing to apply a few simple habits that I will highlight in the coming pages.

What will this book do for you?

This book will provide you with motivation, tips and advice to get and stay active. It will give you the exercises and nutrition advice as well as many other key elements that are needed to raise the bar at 50 and older.

What else is coming in the book?

I have trained hundreds of people over my fourteen-year career as a fitness trainer. This book will give you stories and insights into the health and wellness journeys of people that I handpicked to inspire you.

I will highlight and bust some key myths that might be stopping you from receiving results. Raising the Bar is also filled with some of the best exercises to perform, and my top foods for you to eat. Also included is a sample workout plan for beginners.

L.T. Thomas

Chapter Two:
Who am I & The Purpose of this book

"Efforts and courage are not enough without purpose and direction."
John F. Kennedy

Who am I?

As a young kid I always had a love for being active. My parents fueled this drive by enrolling me in sports at the age of seven. In high school I was a three-sport athlete. I played football, track & field and I wrestled. I realized my passion to be a fitness trainer in the 10th grade. I made up my mind that I was going to pursue a fitness degree in exercise science. Before starting college, I decided to join the army reserves. The challenge of basic training interested me in this journey. This was a great experience that challenged me physically as well as mentally. After finishing basic training, I was off to college. I graduated from Salisbury University with a bachelor's degree in Exercise Science. Finishing school was a great feeling, but little did I know it was just the start of my learning journey.

Here are some of my other fitness and education highlights:
- Owned a Personal Training Studio
- Owned a Fitness Boot Camp Studio
- Managed a Team of Trainer at a Commercial Gym
- Fitness Podcaster
- Form Member of USA Army Reserve
- Graduate Certificate in Management and Leadership – Liberty University
- Completed National Academy of Sport Medicine Personal Training Certification
- Primal Health Coach – in progress
- Ace Health Coach Certification
- CanFit Pro Personal Training Specialist
- TRX (Total Body Resistance Exercise) Suspension Group Training Qualification
- DTS Level 1 Specialist (assessments to advance program design)
- DTS Mobility Stretching

- DTS Lean Body Fat Loss Coach
- Fitness Boxing Institute

Why did I write this book?

I decided to write this book because it motivates me to see anyone working out, especially people that are older than me. When I see him or her exercising, it makes me want to work out as well. My goal is to be fifty and active one day. I look up to and admire people that are doing it now. The respect that I have for them is what inspired me to write this book. Working out in itself is hard enough at any age. As you age it doesn't get any easier, but it sure does help to keep you feeling younger.

Working out is a great way to increase your energy level. It allows you to get through the day without being exhausted. It even relieves stress. Completing workouts gives you a sense of accomplishment. It empowers you to want to do more. It elevates your mental clarity and it increases your focus. I hope this book energizes you to want to exercise, empowers you from the knowledge and stories in this book, and elevates you to a better quality of life.

I have been blessed to meet a number of different people that are working out on a regular basis at 50 and older. It's never too late to start and you are never too old to continue. So, I pray that this book will be a blessing to people of all ages and sizes because all of us need to exercise.

I have interviewed people of all levels. Some are very fit, and others have only been working out for less than a year. I have also interviewed people that love working out and others that can't stand it but know it's a must. No matter your current fitness level, there is a story in this book that I am certain will benefit you.

> **Myth: If I am not sore the next day, then I didn't work out hard enough.** You shouldn't be sore after every workout. If you are always sore, then you are probably not recovering enough, or you are exercising too much. A fitness trainer can help you balance this out.

Chapter Three

The Stories

"Stories can empower you or deflate you."

Lemuel B. Thomas Jr.

Raising the Bar Stories

The following stories came from my actual clients. As I was noticing their fitness levels rising, I was getting more inspired to learn their secrets and pass them on to others. So, I created a simple survey and asked some of my over-50 clients to respond. Here's what they told me.

Deb Stratas, age 58

I have enjoyed a forty-year career with IBM – mainly as a Senior Learning Designer. I love to create learning programs that help leaders be more effective. And I've had the good fortune to have influenced thousands of IBMers and traveled to many international locations.

I'm also a published author – having written two novels about Princess Diana. I truly enjoy the historical research and bringing the late Princess of Wales back to life in fictional form.

I live in a suburb of Toronto, Canada.

Why did you get started working out?
I started working out because I felt I wanted to get more fit and healthy as I got older.

How did you get started?
I started working out a local gym with my teenage daughter. We used to do classes together – aerobics, step, Pilates, etc. I loved those classes!

How long have you been working out?
About 15 years on a regular basis.

What is your favorite workout activity?
Wow, that's hard to say. I love changing things up and doing different activities. I always like weight training – it makes me feel strong. I still love group classes, but I have to be careful about anything high impact because of arthritis in my knees. I still like aerobics and circuit videos, though. Being outside is also great – riding my bike on the nature trail near my house and yoga in the park are favorite pastimes.

What do you struggle with as it relates to living a healthy life style?
I have to confess that my biggest guilty pleasure is dark chocolate. I try to limit myself to 2 squares a day but I could easily eat more. Just offer it to me!

What motivates you to continue to work out?
I will be retiring soon, and I see it as the next, exciting chapter in my life. So, I want to be as fit and strong as possible. I want to live a long and active life. I want to spend as much time as possible with my kids and my grand-daughter. Also, my father has health problems (diabetes, heart issues) that I want to avoid, if at all possible.

Why is working out important to you?
I want to feel strong and fit and healthy. And I want to continue to travel and be very active in retirement.

What does your workout routine consist of?
Right now, I'm working with LT as a personal trainer twice a week. He puts me through a thorough body workout, including lots of core work, weights and other strength exercises. I also bike ride and do cardio on off days. And I love to walk whenever I can.

What advice would you give to others about working out and being healthy?

I would say that you don't have to start out with a big commitment (e.g. xx amount of weight loss or even working out xx times per week). Just get started – pick an activity you love and increase steadily from there. Once you start to feel good, it motivates you to do more!

How has working out and eating healthy affected your life?

Here's a perfect story to answer this question. I recently returned from a very busy trip to London, England. After having lost twenty-five pounds and amping up my workout routine this spring and summer, I feel great and much more energetic. I was easily able to handle all the rigors of travel, including walking for at least 3-4 hours a day to visit the sites I really wanted to see. Even six months ago, I would have been more tired, had to take more breaks and possibly even omitted certain destinations because they would have been too tiring. Can't wait for my next trip!

> *Myth: Brown rice is healthy.* It's a little healthier than white rice, but not by much.

Wendy Moran, age 56
Pickering, Ontario
Grew up in Toronto and went to University of Toronto
I graduated with Honors, with a Bachelor of Arts in French Language and Translation.
Currently a Project Manager at Canada's Largest Printing Company in Toronto

Why did you get started working out?
Unemployed, and feeling incredibly depressed about it, I had a gym membership so used this as a reason to get out of bed in the morning and met LT, the trainer.

How did you get started?
I got started with a trainer at GoodLife. He believed in me and encouraged me and through his positive attitude, I stuck with it.

How long have you been working out?
Just over 2 years.

What is your favorite workout activity?
Strength training.

What do you struggle with as it relates to living a healthy life style?
Breaking bad eating habits in the evening.

What motivates you to continue to workout?
I'm 55 (56 tomorrow) and want to be flexible and mobile as I age. I also like my new body and like the new extra energy I have.

Why is working out important to you?
Plus, it puts me in a great mood. If I've had a bad day at work, then I can run off steam. No matter how I feel

when I get to the gym, I feel fantastic when I leave. Mood stability, emotional happiness - much improved.

What does your workout routine consist of?
I attend Boot camp twice a week, plus cardio/stretching/strength once or twice at the local gym. I like the outdoors so spend time outside walking/hiking.

What advice would you give to others about working out and being healthy?
Once you get past the hurdle of getting started, once you realize no one is looking at you and judging you, once you believe you can be successful, it gets a lot easier.

How has working out and eating healthy affected your life?
It has improved it immensely. Working out helps me to sleep better, helps with menopausal mood swings and dealing with a stressful life. Eating healthy has affected my measurements, weight, skin, mood, energy levels; and digestive issues are a thing of the past. I was on high blood pressure meds but since I've lost 50+ pounds, I don't need them anymore. I have better self-esteem. Since a (wonderful) trainer has believed in me, I've been able to believe in myself. I have more confidence than I've ever had.

Myth: Eating fat will make you fat. This depends on the type of fats. You have healthy fats and you have unhealthy fats. *Good fats:* olive oil, coconut oil, avocado butter, the whole egg. *Bad fats:* soya/soybean oil, canola oil, vegetable oil, margarine.

Joanne Waite, age 54

Bio - married, 2 adult children. I Completed College Diploma and University Certificates. Currently I am pursuing University Undergraduate Degree.

Hometown is Ajax.

I am a Retired Police Officer.

Started working out regularly after retirement as I felt that I was in the worst physical condition of my life. I wanted to be able to fully enjoy retirement and having a higher level of fitness and feeling more comfortable would benefit my goal.

I tried to work out on my own initially as I had worked out many years earlier and had a pretty good idea of how to properly lift weights. However, I couldn't get into a routine. I felt that I needed someone to push me a bit and keep me in check, so I looked into finding a trainer.

I have worked out off and on over the years. Early in my career it was necessary for me to have a specific level of fitness, but maintaining that level consistently was a battle with shift work and the responsibilities of raising a family. This current round I have been working out for about 6 months.

My favorite workout activity is muscular strength and endurance training. I enjoy lifting weights. But I also enjoy variety and the comradeship of team sports especially ice hockey.

When I worked, I used to struggle with getting proper sleep/rest. I felt exhausted often which also made regular workouts difficult. But I have always and still do struggle with getting enough cardiovascular exercise. I find cardio work to be boring.

I am motivated to continue workouts because I want to feel great and I want to look fabulous. I want my husband to always be attracted to me on the outside, not just the inside. I see a lot of women who let themselves go. I don't want to be one of them.

My workout routine consists of muscular strength and endurance training 2 - 3 times a week, walking and stretching on most days, then a variety of different activities to keep me moving; anything from ice hockey, to bicycle riding, swimming or gardening. I need to find ways to incorporate more cardio exercise.

Advice to others: Little bits add up to a lot. Don't feel you need to start off with a routine that bogs you down. Doing anything is better than nothing. It's about making changes that are sustainable in your life. And if you fall off the wagon, pick yourself up the next day and get back on...it's not failure, it's just part of the journey.

Working out and eating healthy has me feeling better as a whole. I have more energy and I feel stronger. As I see changes in my body, I feel good and that is motivating to do more. And when I get a compliment, I feel great!!

Myth: Lifting weights doesn't help with weight loss. Lifting is a great way to assist in weight loss because of the number of calories that you burn and the hormone response.

Lorraine N Bergkvist Baltimore, MD, age 67

I currently live in Baltimore City and I am 67 years old. The highlights of my career include running a computer consulting firm and teaching middle school science. I have a bachelor's degree from Trinity University and a master's from Towson University. I have three children and seven grandchildren. Presently, I am a professor at the University of Baltimore and also a resume consultant for folks looking for new jobs. I run the business from my home. In addition, I am a professional singer.

Athletics have been an important part of my life as long as I can remember. I won an award in high school for athleticism and got to visit the Military Academy at West Point, NY along with the captain of the football team who won for the boys. Back in those days we didn't have sports events for girls. The gym teachers chose me. I had distinguished myself by playing in a county-wide badminton tournament.

I was quite nimble at badminton because my father used to run a Parks and Rec badminton league in the fall and winter in New York for his buddies when I was in high school. Often, they needed a sub so I played regularly. Currently, I occasionally play in UB's badminton intramural program. I can beat most players except the small Asian women who hardly let me earn a point.

My favorite sport is tennis. My dad was a tennis-pro so my sisters and I had to learn. He only gave up the game two years ago when his vision became too impaired. He is 96 and calls tennis a life-time sport.

Since then, I have always played tennis but only began playing year-round when my children were grown. Now I play 3 to 4 times a week with organized groups or on a USTA team. I haven't signed up for the senior division yet because my daughter captains several teams and still asks me to participate with her.

My other favorite sport is bike riding. Since I moved to the city, I ride very often. I find it easier to get around the downtown area for shopping, banking, or to work on a bike. I even ride in the rain but not below 40 degrees. I have been on three multi-week European bike trips (around southern France, Berlin to Prague, and a barge and bike trip up the Seine to Paris) and one through the Outerbanks.

I started strength training about 3 years ago. I stopped working full-time and I moved to the city I found the gym convenient. In the country, you always have to take a car to get somewhere. I noticed older ladies among my bridge acquaintances had instances of falling. When they did, they broke something, and their health went downhill from there. I am determined to build up some muscle mass to protect my bones and joints.

I chose the MAC gym because my husband liked the pools the best. I liked the convenience because I will not drive to get there. I don't really like working out, but I know it's necessary. It's easiest when I have sessions with my personal trainer.

I struggle with weight control and that is a strong incentive for me to keep working out. I am about 19 pounds over my Weight Watchers goal. My specific routine includes riding my bike to and from the gym and carrying out activities recommended by my trainer. I try to do this twice a week – once with him and once alone. I want to be able to handle it on my own. It is a struggle to maintain the schedule because of my professional obligations. I do quite a variety leg, core, and arm activities – many on the machines. My favorite activity is stretching at the end of a session.

My advice to others is to make working-out/athletic activities at least as important as your job. It becomes even more essential the older you are. I think it keeps me thin, healthy, energetic, and gives me a great night's sleep.

> *Myth: Sports drinks are good for you.* Sports drinks are usually very high in sugar, so they should be avoided.

Cindy Macdonald, age 77

Born in 1941, I have a degree in English from Bates College, Lewiston, Maine, a Master of Arts in Teaching degree from Harvard Graduate School of Education in Cambridge, Massachusetts, and a Masters in Administration and Supervision from Northeastern in Illinois. I grew up in Springfield, Massachusetts, and lived in Germany, Rhode Island, New Jersey, and Chicago (for 32 years), before moving to Baltimore in 2006. I'm a retired high school teacher /administrator and college instructor.

Why did you get started working out?

I had read that lifting weights was essential to staying strong and flexible and for preventing bone loss. I also read that if I lift weights my body would continue to burn more calories even when I sleep. That works for me, multitasking while asleep!

How did you get started?

My parents had always walked, often taking us kids with them, so as an adult I often walked, but not systematically. When I approached fifty, I saw an aerobic step for sale on TV, so I bought it, and immediately perceived that my body was working much harder when I used the step than with just walking. I think a resistance cord came with it, so I started to use that as well. And then I started to read about fitness.

How long have you been working out?

For 20 years or so I've tried to incorporate aerobic activity and weights into my routine, but I've done different things at different times, and sometimes, more often than I'd like to admit, I've done pretty much nothing, Over the years I've had a couple of different gym memberships and belong to one now. I've been fairly consistent for about four years and have recently engaged a personal trainer to get the most out of my time and effort.

What is your favorite workout activity?

I like different activities, but probably my favorite is dumbbells. I like the fact that I'm exercising many muscles at once as I stabilize the weight. Once again, I'm basically lazy, so multitasking works.

What do you struggle with as it relates to living a healthy life style?

I have a sweet tooth and I love to read. Added together, that leads to an inactive life style. I have to be intentional about moving around and eating vegetables or a healthy life style won't happen.

What motivates you to continue to work out?

I don't want to buy a whole new bigger wardrobe, I like to be strong and flexible, and my body actually feels better overall when I work out. Also years ago I met a woman who had just turned 70 and was training to participate in a triathlon. I bring her to mind when I think I'm too old to be doing this.

Why is working out important to you?

I belong to a continuing learning community which consists of vitally engaged people, mostly over 70, many over 80, so weekly I see the necessity of continuing to exercise one's body as well as one's brain. It's easy to tell which folk are active, and though some who have been active are infirm now, that is a further reason to try to stay strong as long as possible.

What does your workout routine consist of?

For about four years I have worn a pedometer almost daily and it motivates me to aim toward walking four miles a day. Even though I may fall far short, I have a constant reminder to try to avoid low numbers. About two or three times a week, if the weather permits, and it usually does, I walk to the gym, a distance of a little over a mile. I lift weights, swim, and walk home again. At the gym I do six exercises, three sets of 10 or 12 repetitions each for a total of 18 sets. I do all the sets for two exercises before moving on to the next two. It takes under half an hour total. If I can't get to the gym for some reason, I still have my old eight-inch step and resistance cord, which I use, or I do some yoga routines from my WII Fit.

What advice would you give to others about working out and being healthy?

Just do it. You can start easy by moving around more and lifting soup cans. If you don't work out for a time, don't be discouraged and quit. Start up again. It all helps to keep you healthy. So many diseases and so much infirmity are tied to a sedentary life style. It's hard to get started and it does take time, but it's worth it

How has working out and eating healthy affected your life?

I've always had trouble keeping my weight down, but the more weight I carry the more trouble I have with pain in my back and legs due to spinal stenosis. Healthy habits therefore keep me feeling better. Also, I've had scary bouts with cancer and a twisted intestine. Some things I have no control over, but I realize I have a responsibility to do the best I can by making healthy choices. We moved to Baltimore to be with our grandchildren, and I'd like to be with them as long as possible and to take part in their activities. I even surprised myself by going horseback riding with my granddaughter the other day. I'm stronger now than when I was when I was younger, and it feels good.

Myth: To lose the fat around your stomach, you need to only do abdominal exercises. Abdominal exercises alone will not burn enough calories to flatten your stomach. It's more about what you are eating. Decreasing the carbohydrates and the insulin response to

---

enable your body to burn more fat instead of carbohydrates.

Timothy Twomey, age 60

I am a lawyer and architect, currently practicing law as deputy general counsel in a large, international architectural and engineering firm headquartered here in Baltimore and with offices across the US and in England, China and the Middle East. I have a BS in Architecture from the University of Southern California, a law degree from UCLA, and a Masters in Architecture from Harvard University. I was born and raised in West Los Angels, and have lived for the past 35 years in Providence, Rhode Island, Boston, Massachusetts, and now in Baltimore, Maryland.

Why did you get started working out?

I wanted to improve my overall health, lower my blood pressure, reduce my cholesterol, and reduce my weight.

How did you get started?

I signed up at MAC after checking a couple of other places.

How long have you been working out?

About five weeks now.

What is your favorite workout activity?

No favorite - enjoy the weights, the treadmill and the stationary bicycle.

What do you struggle with as it relates to living a healthy life style?

I eat too much, and too much of the wrong foods.

What motivates you to continue to workout?

The same reasons that got me started - improve my overall health, lower my blood pressure, reduce my cholesterol, and reduce my weight.

Why is working out important to you?

It provides a structure for exercising, a routine that makes it easier to exercise.

What does your workout routine consist of?
Two days a week on weights, and two days a week doing cardio. The days alternate.

What advice would you give to others about working out and being healthy?
Do it. It's good for you. You'll feel better for doing it.

How has working out and eating healthy affected your life?
I'm still working on the eating healthy part but working out makes me less fatigued in regular daily activities and is strengthening my legs which I feel is needed. By eating healthy I'll lose weight and that will also help with strengthening my legs. Working out is also lowering my blood pressure.

Myth: Squats are bad for you. Squats are probably the best exercise because they involve all your major muscles to perform.

Sue Panther, age 50
Education: MAEd in Literacy from Eastern WA University in 2000
Hometown: I've resided in Spokane, WA for the past 25 years, but I was born in Seattle, WA

Current Position: Certified substitute teacher middle school and high school English/Language Arts and reading; substitute teacher Spokane College of English Language; online writing TA Ashford University.

Why did you get started working out?
I've always valued fitness; aerobics became the fad when I was a freshman in college. I was a swimmer in high school, so it made sense to continue that in college as well; then I got hooked on intramural crew and, of course, running.

How did you get started? In high school I joined the swim team. In college, I dated a guy who was a cross-country runner, so he got me hooked on running.

How long have you been working out? I've been working out all of my adult life, so GASP over 30 years.

What is your favorite workout activity?
I am obsessed with running. The people in my neighborhood who don't know my name just call me "the runner." They even come up to me at the mall or the grocery store and say, "Hey, I see you running past my house all the time."

What do you struggle with as it relates to living a healthy life style?
I don't have quite the stamina I used to, and as a single mom, it can be a challenge to find the time, motivation and energy to have a true, consistent workout schedule.

What motivates you to continue to workout? I have a 7-year old daughter so I need to stay fit and healthy to keep up with her; Also, I have always cared and WILL always care about how I look. I don't want to see an old, out of shape woman when I look in the mirror.

Why is working out important to you?
It helps me reduce stress, look good, feel more energetic, and my runs and time at the gym are about the only time I have to myself.

What does your workout routine consist of? I alternate between running 4-6 miles (I also alternate between steady runs and interval training); lap swimming for 45 min - an hour, and cardio and strength training (a 2-mile warm up on the treadmill or elliptical, then strength training, followed by a 1 mile cool down either on the treadmill or the spin bike). When I am in training for triathlons I cut back on the weights and spend more time on my road bike.

What advice would you give to others about working out and being healthy?
Make staying healthy a priority; schedule workouts like you would any other appointment; find a workout buddy to help with motivation - if you commit to walking, running, meeting at the gym you're more likely to go so you don't stand up your partner than if it's just about you. As far as eating right, don't look at food as your enemy. You need good nutrition, flavor, color...ENJOY your food, don't just eat to eat. And don't eat mindlessly. NEVER eat in front of the tv or on the fly. If you savor your food, you are less likely to overeat. Also, be aware of what you're putting into your body. Processed foods, preservatives, hormones and all things that come via a drive-thru window are likely what's sabotaging your efforts to maintain a healthy body weight (and a healthy body). Eat more unprocessed foods

(fruits, vegetables, fish, chicken, eggs, greek yogurt) and less sugar, white flour, pre-packaged snacks...

How has working out and eating healthy affected your life?

I have people remark all the time that I don't look 50, and I definitely don't feel my age. I am able to do all the things I want to do including road races, triathlons, outdoor activities, play on the jungle gym with my youngest daughter. I hope to continue to workout and stay fit for decades to come!

Myth: You should hit the gym every day. If you work out every day your body will not recover. So, you will limit your results and possibly injure yourself. Only low-level activity should be done every day: walking, hiking, biking, stretching.

Mary M. Williams, age 60
Education: College of New Rochelle, BSN
Hometown: Garnerville, NY
Current Position: Registered Nurse

Why did you get started working out?
To get stronger, healthier and stay shapely.

How did you get started?
After I got married i started gaining weight and didn't like the way I was starting to look.

How long have you been working out?
I started working out since I was about 23-24 years old and now at the age of 60 i am training harder than I've ever been.

What is your favorite workout activity?
Just about any exercise that keeps me in shape including weight training.

What do you struggle with as it relates to living a healthy life style?
Not much. I try to eat foods that are beneficial to healthy living.

What motivates you to continue to workout? I want to maintain a healthy life style and to stay within a certain size.

Why is working out important to you? It keeps my mind focused on staying healthy and I interact with people who want the same things.

What does your workout routine consist of?
Cardio and weights: Spin cycle, treadmill, elliptical and Stairmaster. I'm also able to afford a personal trainer to keep me focused.

What advice would you give to others about working out and being healthy? Exercise at least every other day in some form and try to eat foods that are good for the body. Cut out sugars and extra salt, maintain a balance diet and eat small portions. Drink plenty of water especially before each meal.

How has working out and eating healthy affected your life?
It helps me to look and feel very good about myself.

Myth: Sit ups are the best exercise for your stomach. Sit ups involve your quads as well as your hip flexors, so it is not a good exercise to target your stomach. Planks are the best exercise for your core and stomach.

Thomas Stewart, age 49
Why did you get started working out?
Earlier in life, I worked out because I enjoyed competing. Basketball and running were the sports I enjoyed playing the most. Around the age 38 I stopped playing basketball because of all the nagging injuries. I ran sporadically during this period, but I decided after my first child was born when I turned 44 that I should pursue running again.

I now run less for competition sake and more so that I can keep-up with my five-year-old who, ironically, loves to run. Now, that I have a second child at the age of 49, it is extremely important to me to maintain great health and modeled for my children the importance and value you of great health.

How did you get started?
Because I have a history of running that is over 25 years old, it comes very natural for me. However, I had to make a stronger commitment to weight training, stretching and other works outs that don't involve running. I currently run 2 to 3 days a week, and I bike, swim and/or do yoga at least two other days. I found it very important to work out with a training for a few sessions to identify the appropriate exercises given my goals and objectives.

How long have you been working out?
Over 30 years.

What is your favorite workout activity?
Running, swimming, weight training, yoga and biking (in that order).

What do you struggle with as it relates to living a healthy life style?
Ideally, I would like to devote 90-120 minutes for each work out at least four days a week. Given the other

demands on my schedule, maintaining consistent work outs is my greatest challenge.

I am motivated by the confidence and peace of mind being health gives me. Also, knowing that good health will allow me to enjoy my two young children is a huge incentive.

What advice would you give to others about working out and being healthy?

Exercise can sometimes seem like a very selfish thing to do. However, the reality is that maintaining good to excellent healthy is the best gift you can give the people you love. Most people who are committed to working out are far less likely to engage destructive behaviors (gambling, eating disorders, alcoholism substance abuse, etc.).

They are also more likely to have time and energy for the people that matter most. Make working out something you do as part of your lifestyle. It might be difficult at first to do it consistently, but once you make it a priority and incorporate it into your life it will become second nature.

How has working out and eating healthy affected your life?

Though I will turn 50 my next birthday, I am often told that I look 40. That says it all....

Myth: You can turn fat into muscle: Your body burns fat and build muscle, but fat is not going to turn into muscle.

Karen Parker, age 62
Currently Resides in Oshawa
Hometown Saint John New buckwick
Retired from Law enforcement with Toronto Housing

Why did you get started working out?
I had been trying for a few years to work out but never stuck to it, for one reason or another.

How did you get started?
I decided to use a personal trainer instead of going to the YMCA as I done in the past, which I didn't stick to.

How long have you been working out?
I have been going to work out twice a week with my personal trainer for just over 3 months regularly.
Before this, I worked out off and on throughout the years but never really stick to it. When I was much young, I was very active in basketball as well as track and field.

What is your favorite workout activity?
I enjoy TRX Pull ups, the leg press machine, and the sled.

What do you struggle with as it relate to living a healthy life style?
I struggle with the paleo diet, not that I'm cheating. Making time for cooking has been the toughest part for me. I have been out of the habit of cooking regularly for the last few years.

What motivates you to continue to workout?
I have been feeling a lot better and have more energy then I use to have.
Why is working out important to you?
It is very important for me, at my age to be more active.

What does your workout routine consist of?

I perform weight training twice per week as well as regular walking throughout the week.

What advice would you give to others about working out and being healthy?
I would advise people to start early in life and stick to it. That is eating healthy and exercising.

How has working out and eating healthy affected your life?
I feel so much better, and stand straighter, I also enjoy working with LT, he made sure that the exercises I do won't affect my disabilities, my back and my knees. I am not sore the next day, like I had been in the past when I exercised.

Changing the way I eat has been a big improvement for me, besides eating more vegetables and fruits; I feel my diet helps with my diabetes as my numbers have been in my target range since I started eating better.

One thing I hope to do while working with LT is to stop using the cane, I have been using, since 2006. When I achieve that, I will know that I made the right decision to work with a personal trainer. I only wish I started sooner.

Kevin Corless, age 58
Education: RCSI med school in Dublin Ireland
Hometown: Ireland
Current Position: Medical Doctor

I currently live with my wife and family in Oshawa, Ontario. I am a Med Director of The North Oshawa Med Center. I was born in Chicago III USA on May 6, 1960. I played grade school American football till age 12 when my family moved to Ireland where my parents were from.

I played High school rugby and soccer and continued playing both during med school until 1985 when I graduated from RCSI med school in Dublin Ireland.

I met my wife while working at a summer job in Toronto and immigrated to Canada in 1987. I played soccer and rugby for a few years and then mainly squash during my family years. With 7 kids there was not a lot of free time to play and commit to organized sports.

In recent years I took up golf and worked out with LT my personal trainer.

I got started 1 year ago when a friend of my daughter advertised, he was a personal trainer and he would make it easier for me to exercise by coming to our house to train me. I got started with a personal trainer because I developed Parkinson's disease and wanted to get fitter than I was and also stretch out against the stiffness of the disease.

My first personal trainer moved away, and my wife found LT on-line and liked what she read, and she made a great   choice
I have been exercising for a year and 3 months. My favorite activity is the "bird dog" as it is not that hard to do but it's harder to maintain the position. I feel like I'm using all my muscles whole performing this exercise.

The hardest healthy lifestyle thing to do is work out on my own.

I keep motivated to work out by the fact that exercise has shown to be so vital of a tool in keeping healthy and both physically and more than ever mentally. It is important for the same reason.

My routine is LT weekly for an hour and doing a routine he lays out for me 2 times a week and swim every day.

My advice to others is "just do it!" Even a small amount of exercise can reduce your risk of heart attack and stroke and you'll look and feel better doing it. Don't make huge plans to work out at the start. Pick a small time to schedule so you know you can achieve it and build up from there.

Lynn McGuire, age 56
Retired IT Bell Canada 35 years

I have worked out on and off most of my life. Most recently I started again when I retired two years ago and now have the time. I work out twice a week with a personal trainer and walk the other 3 days for a minimum of 30 minutes. I find this has helped my mental health, feeling both happy and healthy. I am also sleeping better. My body is more flexible, and I feel stronger.

I also think now about what I'm consuming. I exercise so do I really need these extra calories? I am motivated as I see small changes in my body and feel more confident in my everyday life.

Chapter Four

Survey Summary

"Don't fear failure so much that you refuse to try new things. The saddest summary of a life contains three descriptions: could have, might have, and should have."

Louis E. Boone

Survey Summary
Here are my key observations from the survey results – tips you can use!

- You don't have to start out with a big commitment. Just get started.
- Once you get past the hurdle of getting started and believe you can be successful, it gets a lot easier.
- Doing anything is better than doing nothing. It's about making changes that are sustainable in your life. And if you get off track, pick yourself up the next day and get back on.
- Make working-out/athletic activities at least as important as your job. I think most people put it on the back burner.
- So many diseases and so much infirmity are tied to a sedentary life style. Even a small amount of exercise can reduce your risk of heart attack and stroke and you'll look and feel better doing it.
- Don't look at food as your enemy. You need good nutrition, flavor, color...ENJOY your food, don't just eat to eat.
- Exercise at least every day in some form.
- Working out can seem like a very selfish thing to do. However, the reality is that maintaining good to excellent health is the best gift you can give the people you love. Most people who are committed to working out are far less likely to engage destructive behaviors (gambling, eating disorders, alcoholism substance abuse, etc.).

Chapter Five
LT's Philosophy & FAQ's

"Those who think they have not time for bodily exercise will sooner or later have to find time for illness."

Mark Sisson, **The Primal Blueprint**

L.T.'S PHILOSOPHY &

FREQUENTLY ASKED QUESTIONS

My philosophy when it comes to fitness and living a healthy life is to be active, eat healthy, sleep and recover. You can shortcut your workout by doing a faster workout. You can shortcut your nutrition by paying for a meal planning service, but there is no shortcut to sleeping. It's best to make time for proper sleep. At least 7-8 hours a night.

There are many different philosophies on nutrition. I follow the primal philosophy for nutrition. Primal is not a weight loss diet; it's more of a way of life. Primal eating can be adapted to any goal you may have. When you talk about eating healthy as it relates to primal, it's more about controlling the insulin response of the body. The more carbohydrates and sugar that you consume, the more your body will demand it. The goal of primal eating is to become more of a fat burner instead of a carbohydrate burner. If you consume too many carbohydrates, your body isn't able to burn the fat that you are storing. When considering healthy eating, at the very least you should do these basic things:

1. Eat home-cooked meals as much as possible.
2. Limit your junk food. When you eat out you are at the mercy of whatever they put in the food.
3. Stay away from processed foods. Food processing is any deliberate change in a food that occurs before it's available for you to eat.
4. Finally, decrease your carbohydrate intake.

Here are the core basics of a primal diet:

Eat: fruits and veggies.

Eat: meats, eggs, nut, seeds, and healthy fats.

Avoid: rice, pasta, breads, cereals, added sugar, and trans fats (pretty much all grains).

In moderation: sweet potatoes, quinoa.

It's never too late to start!

There are a number of reasons why someone may start exercising. Some people begin a workout routine because someone close to them works out like their parents or an older sibling. Others might start because of sports in grade school like me. Others might even start working out because of the influence of a husband or wife.

No matter how long you haven't been working out, it's never too late to start.

What do you enjoy?

Finding a favorite activity is a key way to fit fitness into your life. An activity like golf is a great way to stay active. However, it's not enough alone because you aren't doing any resistance training, but it's a great start. And it will keep you active. When you enjoy something, you look forward to doing it; hence you will probably make time for it more often.

The key to starting an activity is finding something that you enjoy. That doesn't mean you should only do the activities that you enjoy, because you want to cover the three basic activities in fitness (strength, endurance, & flexibility). Finding an activity that you enjoy will keep you more motivated and consistent.

Here are the three basic activities:

Weight training or strength training - any activity that is a weight-bearing exercise. Weight Training builds strength so it works your muscles and strengthens your bones. This is important because as you age, you lose muscle starting at age 28 or so. When you lose muscle, you also lose strength. As you lose muscle your bones become more fragile as well. This is why it is important for all adults to weight-train no matter how old. Here are some examples: body weight exercises, free weights (dumb bell, barbells, and kettle bells, cable machines, TRX & weight machines. TRX is an acronym for a suspension-based exercise system is known as a Total Body Resistance Exercise.

Anything that requires your heart rate to stay elevated for 10 minutes or more. Cardio works your heart. The heart is a muscle as well. So, it needs to be worked. Here are a few examples: Biking, running, walking, swimming, and the rowing machine. Swimming and the rowing machine are great as you age because they are low impact on your joints.

Flexibility – Stretches improves your flexibility. As you age, flexibility decreases so it's important to try and stay as flexible as possible. It will decrease the risk of injuries. I aim to stretch daily to keep my body as mobile as possible.

Regular activity
I think that most people struggle with staying consistent. Consistency is the key to living a healthy life style. Consistency doesn't mean your exercise needs to be intense. You just need to be active in some way each and every day. Low level activity everyday like walking is best. I also feel that a lack of knowledge hinders a lot of people from getting started. My advice would be to do some form of activity. Anything is better than nothing at all. Find a partner to team up with. This will help to keep you motivated. If possible, get a few sessions with a professional.

Do I need a trainer?

I feel that everyone could benefit from a trainer in some capacity. If you are able to invest in one, I highly recommend doing so. You will save yourself a lot of wasted time and learn more than you even bargained for. Having a trainer will help you to challenge yourself on a new level than what you are accustomed to. It is easy to underestimate what you are capable of doing. Having a trainer can bring stuff out of you that you didn't even realize you had in you. It's like a student teach relationship. Students go to school and teachers pull the potential out of students. Sometimes it just takes person to believe in another person.

Here are the top reasons to hire a trainer:

- Reduce injury risk – Poor execution of exercises is a common cause of injury.
- Long-term guidance and motivation – The aging process can decrease your motivation towards exercise. A fitness trainer will provide guidance and motivation to keep you going. Having a fitness trainer enables you to focus on the workout rather than the planning.
- They will provide the structure for you. At the start, it is wise to see your trainer more often to keep you on track. If the budget allows, you should give yourself six months with a trainer once or twice per week to give yourself the time to get results, and the understanding of how to work out. Once you learn the basic movement and the system, you can spread your sessions to once every 3-4 weeks.
- You can use these sessions as a review, follow up and adjust your program sessions. Kind of like a check-in just to keep you on track.
- A trainer is a great resource: they can refer you to other specialists like chiropractors, foot specialists, naturopathic medicine massage, and much more.

- Accountability – Having a trainer reminds you of the reasons you decided to exercise. This is great thing because it helps to increase your desire for exercise. Sometimes it is so easy to forget. It will be much harder to find excuses not to go to the gym when your trainer is expecting you.
- Variety and creativity – It is very easy to get bored with exercise if you are doing the same workout all the time. Having a fitness trainer can make exercise a little more fun and interesting.
- Learn the life-long skills – Fitness is a lifelong skill that we all should work at. Most of us work at every other skill but the one that will allow us to enjoy life the most. A fitness trainer can provide you with knowledge, resources, guidance, training and skills so that you can apply them to a life of fitness.

How do I know a good one?
The first thing you should do is setup a consultation with a fitness professional. Ensure that you get along. If you don't mesh with the trainer it's probably best to find someone that you mesh with. Secondly make sure they are certified. It would be even better if they have a diploma or degree in fitness or something related. Also, the number of years as a trainer makes a big difference. The more experience the fitness trainer has the better. Finally, I would want a trainer that is living what they preach. They should at least look healthy. The trainer doesn't need to look like an elite athlete, but they should be in decent physical condition. This is not a requirement to become a fitness trainer, but it probably should be one.

If you aren't able to hire a fitness trainer, maybe hiring a health coach could be a good option for you. Having a health coach could be a little more cost effective than hiring a fitness trainer. You could meet with the health coach once a month or even biweekly. They can help you stay on track and help with healthy lifestyle habits. This would be a great option to have someone to be accountable to. The great thing about having a health coach is the flexibility. You could do your sessions in person, over the phone, or through video calls. Having a health coach is similar to having a financial advisor. They provide you with the best options for your situation and provide support along the way.

Take your time

Take your time with exercise and gradually progress. Most people's workout routines are not basic enough at the start. I notice that when people take a break from exercise, they try to return back to the same level they were at before they stopped. Fitness is a journey so it's going to be a process. It's going to take time, but it shouldn't be something that you rush because it can cause unnecessary injuries or burn out. You just need to enjoy the process and gradually ease your way into working out and you'll be better off in the long run.

We live in a society that wants everything now, right away. Burger King Slogan sums it up very well "Your Way Right Away." We want fast food, fast weight loss, everything now. The best things are worth waiting for. To get a gourmet meal it's going to take more than five minutes to cook. The same thing is true with a healthy body and a healthy lifestyle. If you want your body to be the best, it's going to take time. If you want to live a healthy life, it's going to take time and effort. One day at a time, one step at a time is the recipe for success. It's not something that can be microwaved. There is no microwave recipe for a healthy lifestyle. The process of creating healthy habits day in and day out consistently is what's going to help you to be healthy.

Fitness equipment suggestions
No equipment is really needed to exercise. However, you can't go wrong with a few pairs of dumb bells. For the

average lady, I would suggest starting off with 8 to 10 lb weight dumbbells. For the average man, I would suggest starting off with 20 lbs. With just a few sets, you can easily have a total body workout. If space is limited, you can simply use bodyweight exercises as well.
Here are my top 5 bodyweight exercises:

1. **Squats**

2. **Lunges**

3. Push Ups
4. Planks
5. Pull ups or invented row (this requires a bar or a trx)

   TRX and a foam roller are my favorite fitness tools. The TRX usually retails for about $150. TRX is an acronym for a suspension-based exercise system and is known as a Total Body Resistance Exercise.

The TRX is a light weight piece of fitness equipment that only weighs about 3lbs. You can do over 20 different exercises with it. It is the ultimate tool for bodyweight training. You can use it in your home and you can take it with you whenever you travel. It is one of my go-to tools that I use when I train clients in their homes. TRX is so versatile that beginners as well as advance exercisers can use it. I even incorporate it into my personal workouts as well.

The next important fitness tool is the foam roller. A foam roller is an exercise device used for massage and fitness. The foam roller is great because it assists your body in recovery. It helps to relax your body and relieve tension. It is also great for improving your posture. If you work at a desk or drive hours per day, it is that much more important for you to have a foam roller.

Chapter Six

LT's Top 10 Exercises &

LT's Top 8 tips for getting started

"It's not only moving that creates new starting points. Sometimes all it takes is a subtle shift in perspective, an opening of the mind, an intentional pause and reset, or a new route to start to see new options and new possibilities."

Kristin Armstrong

Top 10 exercises

Here are my top 10 exercises for people 50 and older:

1. *Squats* are important to maintain strength in the lower body muscles. They are also important to strengthen the knees. Squatting regularly will help you to stay strong enough to stand up and sit down with no problems.
2. *Band or Dumbbell Row:* This exercise is very important to maintaining good posture. Performing a row works your upper back muscles.
3. *Push-ups* are great for the upper body (chest, shoulders, and triceps) but also the core. Since push-ups are a moving plank, they are great to strengthen the lower back and abs.
4. *Dead lifts:* This is my favorite exercise. It works all the posterior muscles (back of thighs, butt, lower back). You can use a kettle bell, dumb bell, or barbell to perform this exercise.
5. *Moving side squat:* It's important to incorporate lateral movements in exercises. Most people focus on going front to back but forget about moving side to side.
6. *Seated twist or Russian twist:* This movement is important because it works on rotation and you are moving in a different plane of motion.
7. *Lunges*: This is great to work on all the lower body muscles as well as balance.
8. *Planks*: This is great for the core but is a total body exercise.
9. *Dead Bug*: This is a great exercise for the core
10. *Bird Dogs*: This is a great exercise for the core and posture.

Top 5 Fitness Websites

Here are my top websites for you to check about fitness, exercise and nutrition:

- LemuelThomasfit.com
- Marksdailyapple.com
- Bodybuilding.com
- Livestrong.com
- fitnessblender.com/

LT's Top 8 tips for getting started:
1. Set a short-term and long-term goal, take pictures, and get measurements so you can chart your progress – numerically and visually.
2. Start with as little as 10 minutes a day.
3. Commit to 2 days a week of strength training and perform low level cardio every day.
4. Mind your nutrition.
5. Listen to your body and allow it to recover.
6. Don't skip on sleep.
7. Walk every day.
8. Have fun! Fitness is a journey so enjoy the process.

What's a good fitness routine?
There are so many fitness routines, but the best one is the one you will actually do! After about 2-3 months of doing the same routine, it's time to change it up. It's best to continue to add variety to your program.

If you are new to working out, I would advise you to work out 2 times per week. Please consult your doctor before starting any fitness program.

Here is a sample program for 2-3 sets of 10-12 reps

This is a total body workout. You are working every major muscle in your body. Be sure to give yourself 1 to 2 days between each workout to allow your body enough time to recover. There are a number of ways to complete this set of exercises. Here is just one example. Repeat each exercise one after another. At the end of the last exercise take a one-minute break.

- Squats
- Push ups
- Bird dogs
- Bands or dumbbell rows
- Dead lifts
- Lunges

Chapter Seven

Final Thought

"Man's greatness consists in his ability to do and the proper application of his powers to things needed to be done."

Frederick Douglass

Final Thoughts

50 and older is a start of a new journey in your life. So, you shouldn't feel like you are too old to make a difference. You still have a lot of life to live. I heard many people tell me that they are too old to exercise. The older you are the more important it is for you to get moving and take care of your health. If you aren't moving on a regular basis, you are slowly **deteriorating**. It's never too late to start living a healthy life. So, get started, be healthy, and have fun.

You *Be*The One

Be means to have the quality of being. *Be* also means someone or something.

You have the quality to *be* special. Everyone is special to someone. Being that you are special, someone loves you. You are someone's mother, father, daughter, son, brother future husband or wife, aunt, mentor, or even role model. No one will care for you like you. Therefore, you *be the one* to care for yourself. You must love yourself before you can fully love anyone else.

There are several meanings of healthy and it means different things to everyone. According to an online dictionary, healthy means having or indicating good health in body or mind; free from infirmity or disease. Being healthy to me means to be able to enjoy life and have fun. It also means, having the ability to be active with family and friends. To go a step further, being healthy even mean that you have decent eating and activity habits. Now, of course, you must enjoy eating but moderation is the key. Eating is definitely one of my favorite activities and Thanksgiving is my favorite holiday, but you must have limitations. You can't just eat any and everything that you like all the time.

It's generally agreed on that 30 days is the time needed to ingrain a new habit. The activity should be performed at least once a day, at about the same time.

You *be* the one to be healthy, first, and foremost, for yourself. *Be* the one to start a workout routine. *Be* the one to cook healthier. *Be* the one to plan healthy activities for your family. *Be* the one to set the trend.

You are not just working out for yourself. You are working out for your kids, your family and your future. Your kids are counting on you. Your future grand-children are counting on you. Your grand-children's kids are counting on you. It only takes one person in a family to start a trend. You *be* the healthy trend starter for your family. Break the trend of obesity. Break the trend of high blood pressure in your family. You are setting an example when you eat healthy and workout. Your kids are watching you. Your nieces and nephews are watching you. You are not only working out for yourself, you are working out for your future. Your workouts could affect generations to come. *Be* the one and set the example. Its starts with you and it starts now. So, *Be the One.*

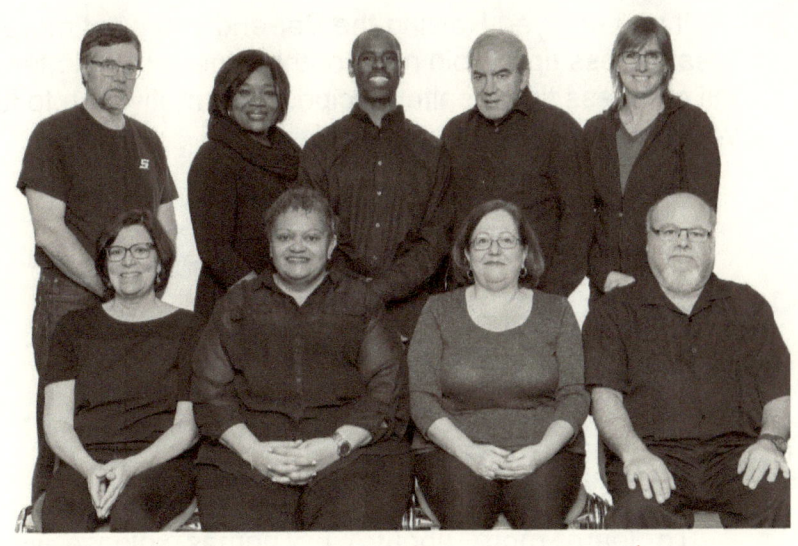

Thank you to my great clients for being a part of this Journey.

Author's Note

If you enjoyed Raising the Bar and you want more great fitness tips. Join my monthly fitness newsletter. It's full of fitness tips, healthy recipes, and motivation to keep you inspired to live a healthy life.

Subscribe at the link below
https://www.lemuelthomasfit.com/subscribe.html

Or

Tune into my podcast
https://www.lemuelthomasfit.com/podcast.html

To learn more about LT Thomas, please visit his website at https://www.lemuelthomasfit.com

You can also follow LT on Instagram @TrainerLT. He'd love to hear from you! LT Thomas

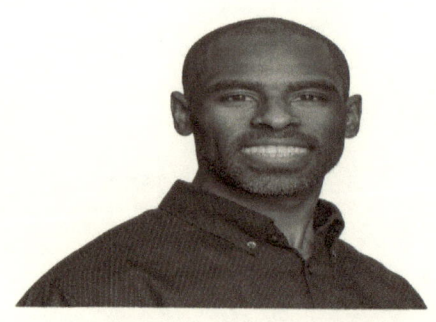

www.ingramcontent.com/pod-product-compliance
Lightning Source LLC
Chambersburg PA
CBHW031328290526
45784CB00014B/2420